# THE GRACE OF
## *Living with Cancer*

## BARB STANLEY, SURVIVOR

"Grace isn't a little prayer you chant before you receive a meal. It is a way to live."

-Jackie Windspear

Balboa Press books may be ordered through booksellers or by contacting:

Balboa Press
A Division of Hay House
1663 Liberty Drive
Bloomington, IN 47403
www.balboapress.com
1-(877) 407-4847

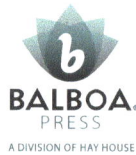

ISBN: 978-1-4525-3606-4 (sc)

Library of Congress Control Number: 2011912234

Printed in the United States of America

Balboa Press rev. date: 7/14/2011

# DEDICATION

This book is dedicated to several angels in my life who have supported me:

- To Pat for sharing the sacred space of your home in the summers to reflect and write my most sacred journey.
- To my husband who has more patience than Job.
- To my children, Christina and Rachelle, who have mentored and taught me more than I EVER taught them.
- To my beloved granddaughters Mia and Danielle, who give me the motivation to LIVE!!
- To my angel friends who have prayed me to this moment in time. You know who you are.

*"The soul at its highest is found like God, but an angel gives a closer idea of Him. That is all an angel is: an idea of God."*

*~ Meister Eckhart*

# BIOGRAPHY

BARB STANLEY was born and raised the town of Red Oak in rural Iowa. She relocated to the metropolitan Phoenix area in 1987. She has worked in the Church in various aspects and is currently teaching at a Catholic high school in Scottsdale, Arizona. She was diagnosed with Chronic Myelogenous Leukemia (CML) in 2002. The following story tells how a cancer diagnosis changed her life—for the better. She hopes to inspire you...

# CONTENTS

# PHILOSOPHY:

How you climb the mountain is just as important as how you get down the mountain. So it is with life, which for many of us becomes one big gigantic test, followed by one big gigantic lesson. In the end, it all comes down to one word: GRACE. It's how you accept the winning and losing, good luck and the bad luck, the darkness and the light.

(This was found on the side of a bottle of Oil of Olay body lotion – with no author to credit. There was only the label that said, "Philosophy 2007.")

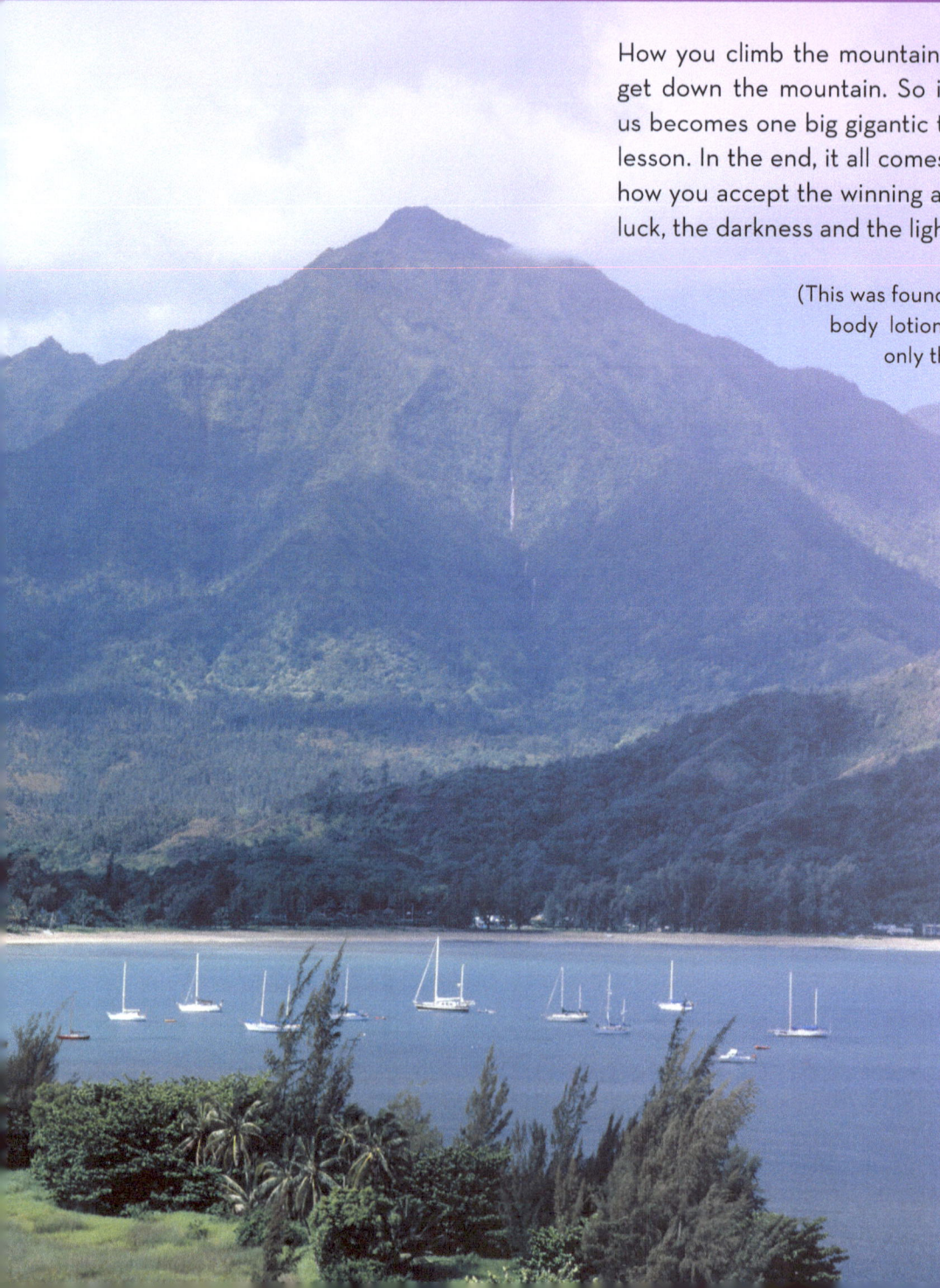

# Chapter 1

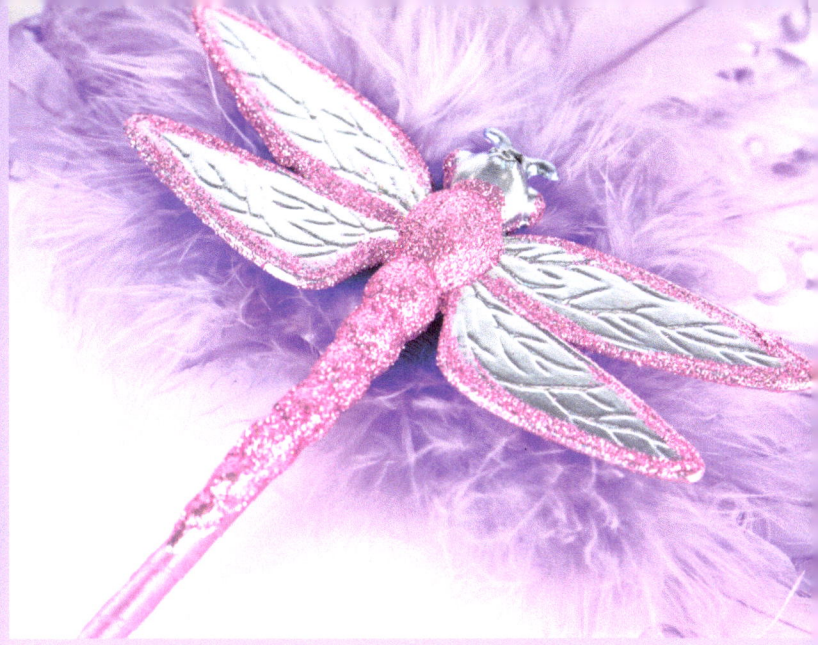

## CHANGE

I am a firm believer that our upbringing, our experiences in our family of origin, and the culture in which we were raised forms the framework for living our lives. Within these contexts, we learn how to make decisions, and we define for ourselves how we will live in relationship with one another. Our *modus operandi* or "MO" is formed, the method of operation for living. Telling you about how I was raised, I believe, will help you understand how I coped with leukemia. It is for this reason that I beg your patience to read a little about my roots.

*When we are no longer able to change a situation, we are challenged to change ourselves.*
*~Victor Frankl*

Being raised in the small Midwestern town of Red Oak of population 5,000 has its good points and its bad points. I always said jokingly that Iowa was "a good place to be *from*," but in all honesty, it truly was. Being raised in the Midwest afforded me the opportunity to live a simple life in a farming community where I could learn the attribute of a hard day's work. Families lived in homogeneous communities where intergenerational child rearing was the norm. Grandma and grandpa lived right up the street. Uncle Jim and Aunt Jean lived nearby and all my cousins went to the same schools and churches. Young people would make one of two different choices. They could marry within the community and work on the family farm or a small business in

*There is always one moment in childhood when the door opens and lets the future in.*
*~Deepak Chopra*

town. The second option was to fly off to the out of state colleges, get their degrees, marry, and settle—to return to the "old home place" only for the Thanksgiving and Christmas holidays. Yes, Iowa was always "good place to come home *to*" also. Things never changed. The trees grew bigger, and the town looked smaller each visit home. The four-lane highway through town seemed to shrink with each visit home. But more importantly, living in the heartland of America helped me to experience the four seasons of the year and the change of each season that was necessary for new life. In Iowa, we were always preparing for the next season. The ground was always prepared for planting in the spring and for harvest in the fall. We would clean out and put in the window air-conditioners in the spring. We covered them up in the fall after we had raked what seemed like millions of leaves. We insulated for winter, and we put new screens on for summer. It was always change in Iowa. The change was good and part of a natural rhythm of the earth and of life. It is this foundation and understanding of change—good change for new life—that carried me through the toughest crises of my life.

The more difficult part of being raised in a small town was the fact that everyone knew everyone else's business. It was so bad that, when someone would lose his job, he would need to hurry home to tell his family before the news got to them "via grapevine." All the traffic tickets, court proceedings, DUIs and speeding tickets, stealing, shoplifting, and divorces made the weekly paper and made for the "top ten" best seller reading list each week. It was usually the neighborhood contest to hurry and read the paper to be the first to call someone and tell her before she had a chance to read it for herself. Adolescents had the entertainment options of a drive-in movie theater, a theater down town, or a house or cornfield beer party. The talk at coffee and donuts after Sunday Mass was always about who had died, who had gotten married, who was having affairs, and who had the latest pregnancy—married or not. You couldn't go to the doctor's office for anything without some small town speculation of what you were there for. The one thing I never missed after we moved was the freedom to live life, tell whom you wanted what you wanted and never have to worry about "What will the neighbors say?"—a constant worry that guided my mother's family relationships and behaviors. She was always afraid that we would somehow embarrass the family.

So after graduation from high school in 1969, I did the small town Midwest thing. I went to beauty school at Americana Academy of Beauty in Des Moines. I got married to a local boy, who went to work for a small business in the farming industry. Neither he nor I had college educations, but we didn't really need them to stay in Red Oak. He was in sales and I was a hairdresser with my own business. I knew everyone in town and everyone knew me. We had two darling daughters who have become the love of my life. We reached "success" as defined by small rural America standards. Life was good.

The word cancer was a familiar word in Red Oak. It still is. A lot of people were diagnosed with various kinds of cancer in the area. It seemed that almost every week the "town grapevine" would announce the most recent death of someone from a cancer diagnosis. (I always thought they should rename our paper *The Grapevine*. As it was, we fondly nicknamed our local paper the Red Oak Excuse instead of the Red Oak Express.) We had industrial companies that were the staple of employment and financial security for the bulk of the town. The plant was located on the banks of the old Nishnabotna River. Our local dump had the means to contaminate this river. That was the same river from which the water was pulled into our treatment plant for our homes. The farming industry required, as usual, using herbicides and pesticides seasonally for treatment of the crops. Of course, in that day and age, no one would dare tell someone not to smoke in any restaurant or home. Myself, I smoked for 17 years, being raised in a home where it was modeled for me as well as being a teen who wanted to "belong." I believe to this day that all of the above factors were a part of the reason that I acquired CML at age 51.

So, success as we defined it, found us in 1987 married, with two girls, one in 7th grade and one in 10th grade, my own salon and with several employees, and my husband selling seed corn for a company out of Nebraska. My oldest daughter was in the middle of her first love with a sweet young boy. My youngest was just entering junior high. Our home, business, marriage, and life were about as good as it could get—at least we thought so. I was involved in church, we had a marriage encounter support group, and we were satisfied. As my husband Bill and I lived out our dream of success, more and more people were moving out of town. This must have been what the "gold rush" felt like in the 1800s. I often thought they should post a sign at the city limits that read, "Would the last one to leave please turn out the lights?" Retired folks were moving to Arizona. Younger families were leaving for bigger and better jobs in bigger cities and in Phoenix. We found ourselves also looking at greener pastures. We had friends who moved to Arizona and made great promises that we could find work if we moved to the Southwest. We debated. As it was, there were 260 houses for sale in a town of 5,000 people. We thought that, even if we decided to move, we would have to take the house payment with us and we were afraid to do that. Bill was more frustrated in his work as the agricultural field really began to struggle. He had held a long desire to go to Arizona. As we talked about it, it became more and more exciting for him—and frightening for me! I had lived within three miles for all thirty-five years of my life. As I became more open to the idea, we put the house on the market and sure enough—after one year, it didn't sell. My husband and I went back and forth. Should we? Shouldn't we? So, I bargained with God. I told God (*like I was I charge?*) if He sold my house, our boat and our car (didn't want to take any payments of any kind with us), that would be the sign we were supposed to go. In one week's time in June of 1987 (mind you, the week after we prayed for a sign from God), not only did the house sell, but so did the boat, and we had a buyer for the car. The final God-inspired message came in the same week, in the form of a job loss: Bill was notified that the family business he had worked for had plans for more family members and no space for him. This has fed my belief that we should really be careful what we pray for—God hears!! It is one of the most important lessons that my Catholic upbringing in the Midwest has taught me: Prayer works!

So we sold all of our belongings, boxed things up and headed south for Mesa, Arizona. Bill had gone on ahead of us, looking for housing and work. He found an apartment based on who would allow our little dachshund puppy. The girls were in tears at leaving their friends, I was in tears at leaving my family, yet, as it all unfolded, and we found the move to be a really good thing for our family. Change once again, was a way for new life. In Red Oak, I had begun to attend classes at a local community college, thinking with great hope that I could indeed, one day, have a college degree. Truth be told, I had secretly admired those peers of mine who went off to college. I just never had the money and didn't think I was college material or that I could learn. The cornfield parties in my adolescence had the effect of putting me on the invite list for the teen social calendar, but ending high school with a graduating 1.6 GPA. I thought college would just be another experience that I would never have.

The girls entered schools in Mesa and got settled, and I took a job as a youth minister at our local church. I began going back to school for theology classes at an institute offered by our diocese. The more I learned, the more I wanted to learn. In my work as a youth minister, I began to "work for the church," and that is where I would remain for the rest of my life. I watched others in the field go back to college and get degrees. The diocese was pushing for education, so I eventually I entered Ottawa University to complete a B.A. in human services. That was such an incredibly good feeling. I found out the good benefits of an education and grew up a little bit while I was at it. I decided to continue my education if I could. I found a great program for a Master's Degree in pastoral theology available summers in Winona, Minnesota. I signed on for the three-year process and spent two weeks each summer and several nights for three years being a college student. Bill had a job working for the City of Mesa. He was secure and stable with it all. I eventually took a job working in an office for youth ministry at the Diocese of Phoenix. Both girls went to college and were out and on their own and life seemed to be once again, stable, and secure. I also entered the third profession of my short time on earth—as a teacher. I remain in this profession today and hope that, it is *the* profession that makes as big of an impact on young people as it has made on me.

By the way, my college GPA was 3.92. You can do anything when you want to.

# Chapter 2

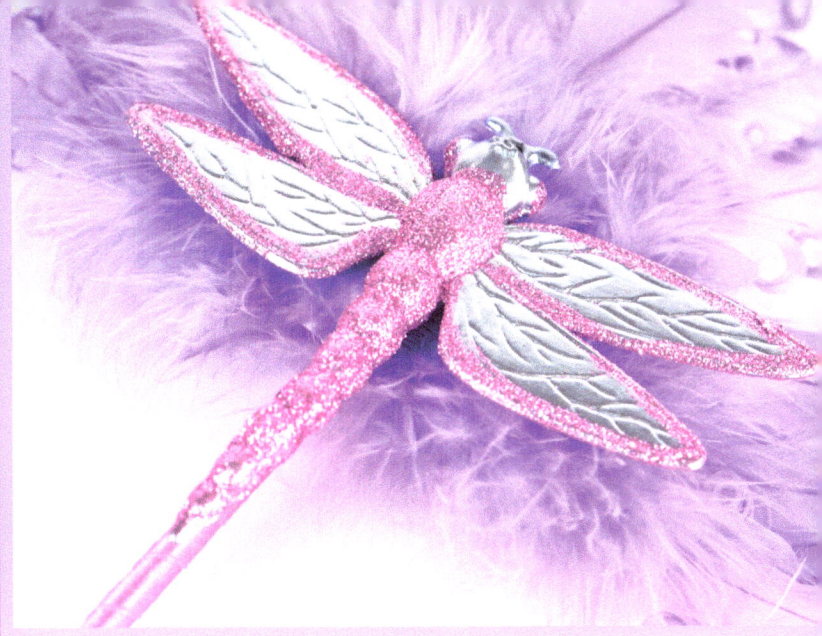

# MOM'S CANCER

Three years after we moved to Arizona, in 1990, my mom was diagnosed with Chronic Lymphocytic Leukemia. Our family was always a family that kept secrets. My mom always thought that she didn't need to worry anyone with details of something we couldn't do anything about, but she would worry herself into a stupor. Consequently, her leukemia was kept from my brother, sister, and me until we stumbled upon a two-week hospital stay that she had the summer of 1993. A good friend of the family called to tell me mom was ill. I flew home that summer and mom sat in the porch swing that now resides on my own back porch, and told me she had Leukemia. After scolding them for keeping

*'Be kinder than necessary, for everyone you meet is fighting some kind of battle.'*
*~T.H. Thompson and John Watson*

this from me for two years, I tried to learn all I could from them. They didn't know much. She assured me that it would not kill her and that it was a condition that she would just have to live with. In my ignorance, I thought somehow the Lymphocytic part of it connected to her chronic bronchitis she had every year and was just one more thing to treat. She was always pretty sickly. She never spoke about the leukemia at all and I never bothered to look up what it was or what it meant. I knew she took medication for it, something called Hydroxeuria. Little did I know that drug was an oral chemotherapy pill I would take myself down the line. Mom didn't talk about it when we visited. She spoke more of her cholesterol, blood pressure, and things that are normally the health issues in older folks. I would ask about the leukemia and she would just tell me it was almost non-existent. I didn't worry much—until one day, in August of 2001, my dad called to tell me that they had discovered a tumor in my mother's liver. There was a hunch that the drugs she had taken for the 11 years she had leukemia had weakened her liver and caused the tumor. It was a fast spreading malignant carcinoma. It was inoperable. They were going to try to treat it with chemo and radiation. In October, she was admitted into a hospital in Omaha, Nebraska, because it was near her oncologist. For my mom, this was the beginning of the end. She was 82. Dad continued to keep me informed while she was in the hospital for several weeks. My brother lived in Des Moines, was single and not really able to come and stay with mom or go to check things out. We had made plans to be back in Iowa the end of October. So when I got there, and checked things out myself, I decided stay on and do what I could.

My arrival home allowed mom to come home. I took a leave of absence for three weeks to stay with and care for her. She was to put on weight and get stronger so she could begin chemotherapy and radiation in a nearby town. They trained us at the hospital to clean out and care for her drain tube they had inserted into her liver, because the tumor was shutting off the bile ducts for proper drainage. It was one of the reasons that she was jaundiced. In all, I had a good three weeks with my mom, and we were able to spend some real quality time and conversation. I had a computer now, and I was on-line, learning all about her kind of leukemia. It was incredibly interesting and frightening at the same time. I left for Arizona and admonished Dad to call me if anything changed in her condition. We left under the premise that Dad would drive her to her chemo and radiation treatments, and that they would plan their first trip in thirteen years down to Arizona as soon as mom finished her treatments the following March.

I returned to Arizona one week before Thanksgiving. My husband and I were planning a celebration in our home, a Mass, and a meal for about 40 people on the Sunday of Thanksgiving week. We were going to renew our

*Being a full-time mother is one of the highest salaried jobs in my field, since the payment is pure love.*
*~Mildred B. Vermont*

vows. November 20, 2001, we would celebrate 30 years of being married. There was a lot to do. I had planned a special surprise to take my husband to Coronado Island in California. He didn't know that I had arranged for his work and all the reservations for a week together. We had never taken a honeymoon. I wanted to really celebrate.

On Thanksgiving Day, we were invited to my daughter's in-laws for dinner. Bill had a turkey on the grill that we were to bring. The phone rang just as the turkey was done. It was my dad. My mom was having signs of her organs shutting down. The ambulance was taking her to the hospital. My brother was there, and Dad said I should come home as soon as possible. I called the girls, and the airlines. God is so good. We found tickets for Omaha for under $200 each. The girls would come with me and Bill would stay in Mesa. We packed and flew to the airport. I was surprised that there were no people there—and then remembered, it was Thanksgiving Day. We flew into Omaha, rented a car, and headed to Red Oak. We walked into the house at 11:30 p.m., my two daughters and me, and collapsed. It was an emotional and long day.

The next morning, we began what would be a four-day vigil until my mother would leave us. She knew me, but was having problems talking. The doctors said the tumor had damaged the liver so much that her other organs were shutting down. They explained that this would be a painful process in which they would keep her comfortable on morphine. Her time would come soon. We stayed in shifts at the hospital as we watched her slip from our presence. On Monday of the following week, mom left us and slipped into the loving arms of our Lord. My oldest daughter was with my mom, while Dad and I were at the house getting cleaned up. Now came the planning of the funeral, the funeral itself, and settling Dad into a new routine. The girls went back home after the funeral and I stayed on to help Dad arrange some personal business. It was December 10 when I finally got back to my own routine.

Since September of 2001, I had had several things begin to affect my health. I had leg pain that seemed to be worse with stress. The night sweats and hot flashes began with a vengeance, I developed insomnia, and had a cold that seemed to hang on and on. I chalked it up to the fact that I would be 51 in April, and decided menopause was moving in with me. They say (I have always wondered who 'they' is!) that a death in the family is a major stress on one's health. I began to lose weight even though I wasn't really trying. Since I believed "them," I chalked up the weight loss and other symptoms to the stress of losing my mom and menopause. I had flown back and forth several times recently, and tried to cope with mom's illness and Dad's fears. People told me that flying so much could cause leg pain. My youngest daughter said that I was looking pretty sickly and that I should go see a doctor. I assured her that I had an appointment the end of April for the well-woman exam. It was the gift I gave myself each year on my birthday month. I knew something wasn't right and I assumed it would be the doctor's decision to put me on medication or hormones for menopause.

# Chapter 3

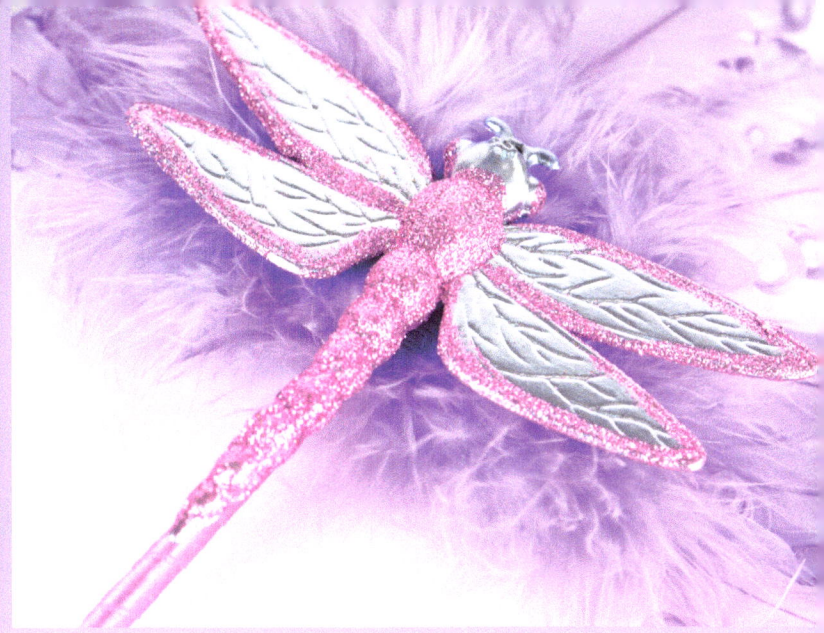

# COURAGE

I had great anticipation of the second half of my life. My girls were out on their own, successful, and happy. I was looking forward to finishing my degree in a little over a year and I longed to work with teenagers again. I was investigating the teaching profession and start a whole new direction in life. There were co-workers who had been encouraging me and I was looking into it. I knew this professional change in my life would be my last. I had been lucky to have three professions in my life that fed my spirit and filled my heart.

It was a little past my 51st birthday that I went to my local family doctor for my yearly well-woman exam. She always insisted on the routine exam to include a pap, a mammogram, blood work, and a general check up. The exam was on a Monday. I told her of my leg pain, my fatigue, the incredibly heavy menstrual cycles and all that had happened in my life in the past six months. She took good notes and ordered all the tests. When I went out the door, I was feeling pretty smug that she would probably call me at the end of the week with a prescription for hormone therapy, I could embrace the entrance into the second half of my life and all would be well. As I went for a manicure, I received a call from my doctor on Friday—but all was not well.

April 17, 2002
Yearly appointment for
Well Woman exam ....
Patient: Barbara Stanley
Doctor: Stacie Schiable
White count: 365,000
Diagnosis?

Leukie has moved in!

As I was parking to see my manicurist, the cell phone rang. My doctor informed me that she wanted to see me. I explained that I was on my way to another appointment and wondered if I could come by afterward. The panic set in immediately. She had NEVER called me like this before. I told her she was scaring me and asked what the problem was. She said that my white count was unusually high and that she had consulted an oncologist. The word "oncologist" told me *cancer*. Then I began to really question her. She informed me that she had a bed already reserved at the Banner Lutheran Hospital for me and that I should go as soon as possible. My blood was compromised in that I had neutropenia—a low neutrophil count. Neutrophils fight off bacterial infections. I was in grave danger of picking up something that could cause my death. Pushing her for more information, Stacy said that I had symptoms of possible leukemia. My heart stopped. I had just buried my mother with leukemia 6 months earlier. I promised to get to the hospital as soon as I could. Then, in a stupor, I went in to get my scheduled manicure. I still do not know why. I think the silly thought went through my head that it isn't nice to cancel an appointment at the last minute. I believe now that it was my short time in denial. I have never been one to spend much time in this space. I finished the manicure, drove home, and called my husband at work. I just told him I needed to pack a bag and head for the hospital. He was home in no time. On the way to the hospital, I took his hand and asked, "Are you ready for this roller coaster ride?" He didn't answer.

They had a bed ready for me all right, and two pages of testing that needed to be done within the next twenty-four hours. I was poked, prodded, jabbed, examined, and X-rayed from every angle. There were promises of more to come in the form of bone marrow biopsies. This was going to be a long haul.

Three days later, my oncologist came to see me to deliver the news. Those were the longest three days of my life. My husband Bill was there as well as my daughter. I tested positive for the Philadelphia Chromosome, which is indicative of CML. I had already been on line with my laptop looking for information and was able to ask about the new drug available for the treatment of CML. He said that would be his first line of defense. He also spoke of the possibility of a bone marrow transplant. I was 51 and the window of opportunity would be closed shortly. I was put on an oral chemotherapy incidentally, the same one my mom was on for CML. I asked him if I could still go to the summer session for my master degree. He said yes but I would need regular blood work every six days while in Minnesota with results being faxed to him within the day of blood draw. I figured I could do that, as long as I didn't miss the summer session. That was the most important thing to me. Cancer would not steal my degree from me.

When the family left, I made phone calls to my best friends, my family members, and my parish priest. The hardest phone call was to my dad. He had just buried his wife and my mother six months earlier. Everything I read said that the life expectancy was three-five years. The new drug was barely a year old and there were no guarantees. I guess the second half of my life was going to look really different to me now.

Then followed the new norm for my life: The constant blood work, the regular bone marrow biopsies, the drug side effects, the fears, and the fight of my life. There was an innate drive within to learn everything I could about CML. I was on the Internet all the time. I bought every book I could about leukemia, transplants, drugs, treatment protocols, and trials. I hooked up with the local City of Hope in Phoenix that was a subsidiary of the City of Hope in Duarte, California. They were at the forefront of transplant protocols. I needed to investigate all of my options. We failed at an attempt to harvest my own cells in case that would be an option down the road. We registered with the National Marrow Donor Program and found two matches: eleven out of twelve. The hematological response to my new drug Gleevec was wonderful.

*"You gain strength, courage and confidence in every experience in which you really stop to look fear in the face. You must do that which you think you cannot do"*
*~ Eleanor Roosevelt*

## Chronic Myelogenous Leukemia

Within nine months, I had reached the ultimate goal: remission. In fact, I have held that remission since. It was a good and hopeful beginning to a dire situation. Since that time, I have switched oncologists, drug protocols, and procedures for treatment of CML—all for the better.

My own possibilities are many, some good and some bad. I could acquire a resistance to the current drug I am on. I could go out of remission at anytime. I could stay in remission for the rest of my life. There are many options out there in the world of leukemia. There are new drugs being developed every day. They are even looking at vaccines for it. If I had to have leukemia, 2002 was a good year to get it.

# Chapter 4

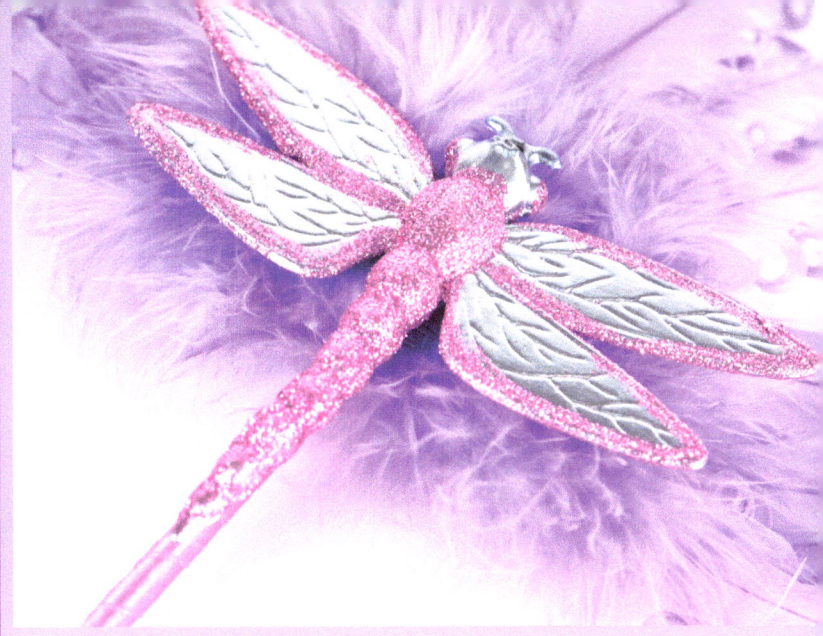

## CHANGE IS INEVITABLE

There is something to "*Change is Inevitable, except from a Vending Machine*" be said about change. It can excite people ~ *Robert C Gallagher* or make them incredibly angry, uncomfortable and stressed. There have been books like "*Who Moved My Cheese?*" explaining the human reaction to change. "Leading Change" is a book that shows ways to guide folks into change in a productive way. My reaction to any kind of change many years ago would have been panic. I see it now as an opportunity to grow.

Growing up in Iowa, we were constantly preparing for change. In the fall, we caulked all the window frames. We raked the leaves and tilled them into the back yard garden. We covered the air conditioner units, fixed broken windows, put on new storm doors, and waited for the cold. In the spring, we would spring clean, open up and air out the house, take all the covers off the air-conditioning units, clean off the coverage of the tulips and crocus, till the garden again, and plant. We trimmed the shrubbery and planted new flowers. The religious significance of dying to new life has always resonated with me. Like the crab apple trees I used to climb in the summer, the old leaves had to die away before the new life could come.

Life's seasons are many. The old ways of life must die away before the new ways of life can emerge. As small children, we are new with life. We are guided by loved ones who help us through our developmental changes. As we grow, we begin the independent task of making our own choices. As a teenager, I was lucky to make it through this stage without any lasting effects on my life. The choices I made were not always good ones. I learned many a good lesson. Even though they didn't become lessons until reflection on my choices as an adult, they are the lessons that guide me today. Painful though the transition from teen to adult was for me, it is has made me a strong person and probably helps me be a good teacher today. At least that is what motivates me to do my best in the classroom. Many a time, I wished I had somewhere to go, someone to talk to. I want to be that person for young people today. I might be older, but the memories of the feelings I had as a teenager are not lessened. Our bodies might change, but our minds and hearts stay with the memories.

I find it very suitable that I contracted CML in the empty nest stage of my life. I believe it was the key to helping me find my direction for the second half of my life. Let me explain.

At one of my employment experiences for a parish in Mesa, the pastor was very big on self-discovery and self-improvement. He not only modeled this for me, but also encouraged me to do the same. He bought books for the staff that were life giving for him. He encouraged us to get counseling when we needed it and even offered to pay for our visits with a Jungian Dream Analyst monthly. In his young wisdom, he recognized the life journey of becoming and tried to influence all those around him with his philosophy. It was in how he treated the staff and the parishioners, and how he related to all the people in his life. I took at advantage of this guiding light.

Mary was an old woman. She was revered in the Jungian community of spiritual directors, and was one of the wisest women I had ever known. On one of the many trips I had to visit with her about my dreams, she made some disturbing comments to me. She implied that I was controlling, that I was spending all my energy in controlling my family and those people around me. I was hurt and angry. I left the place in a huff and vowed never to turn back. After I got over my anger, it occurred to me: She was right. I spent so much energy manipulating others to respond in a manner I thought was correct that I was doing nothing to improve my life—because there was no time. This was the biggest change of all my life. The recognition that I *did not* know it all, do not have all the answers, nor would I ever. Needless to say, I went back to Mary many times after that. She guided me in changing myself, my outlook, my attitudes, and my selfish behavior. It was the best thing that ever happened to me. She made me see change as a series of opportunities in life. With those opportunities, came possibilities for fulfillment and peace. She also taught me this, and I quote her: "You live the first half of your life just living it with not much intention. You live the second half of your life making sense of the first half." I was sure that CML was going to enrich my life but I wasn't sure how.

So the CML diagnosis came and went. As it did, reflection on what this could mean for me became pertinent. I began to journal on this and, to this day, I look back over the entries to remind myself of how far I have come. It was just the change I needed at the perfect time of life. Again, if I had to have CML, 2002 was the best year to get it—for a number of reasons. First, a cancer diagnosis has the possibility of serving as a great springboard for intentional growth in life. I wanted CML to be the opportunity to become wise like my grandmother was wise. This diagnosis was the trigger for self-reflection as I passed into my second half of life.

My grandmother Bruce was the only grandparent I really had a relationship with and it came to me in the 30s of my life. She was a dear woman who worked hard all of her life. She had eleven children and lived to see all but four of them die. She worked the farm as hard as her husband did. Grandma wasn't afraid of anything. She just rolled up her sleeves and did the work because "it needed to be done." When grandpa died and the farm was sold, she moved to Red Oak; thus, began our sacred and blessed time together. I would take her on errands, do her hair, go down for lunch, and take her to church. I was always happy my two girls would know her. I was sure her deep faith would influence them as it had me. She left this world at age 97 having lived by herself until she was 95. She had unconditional love for everyone. She never spoke a cruel or mean word to or about anyone. She was the epitome of unconditional love that my Catholic Christian upbringing had taught me. She became a vital part of my life as an adult and she formed and shaped my philosophy of life. She was the light in my life that helped to define me. For the dysfunctional mother in my life who predicted I would probably not amount to much of anything, my grandma would encourage me with "You will be whatever you wish! Just put your mind to it!" On my 45th birthday, I had my first tattoo. Grandma was long gone, but I decided on a butterfly on my ankle. Grandma had told me that the first half of my life I was the cocoon. The second half of my life, I was the butterfly that brought beauty to people's lives. It was my goal to become what my grandmother predicted. The *change* of living with CML would be perhaps the most important change of my life. But first, I had to get through the rough stuff.

# Chapter 5

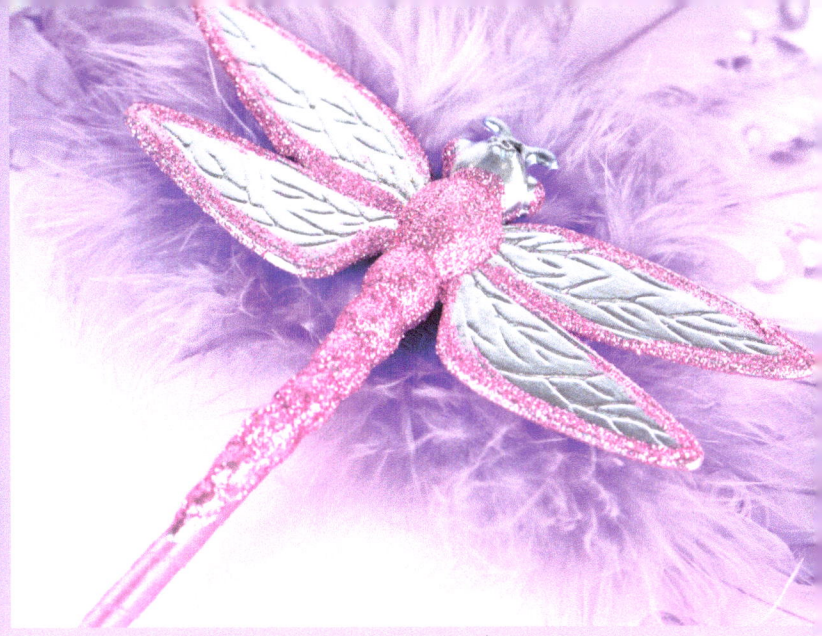

## FEAR

I used to think that grief was only associated with the word *death*. That was until my understanding of death expanded. To me, death is the loss of anything—a relationship, a life, a home, security, and good health. My grandma told me that, each time I fell, I should brush off my knees, get back on the bike, and ride. I didn't want to ride this bicycle. I did not realize that I was grieving the loss of good health until many months after the diagnosis. I am convinced that grief and all of its stages stem from the fear of loss of control. I added the diagnosis information to my life book as another chapter. I just added the information like it was as an addition to the story. I never denied the fact that I had cancer. I did have fears—and felt the need to write them down. Let me share a journal entry that I dated Sunday, May 5, 2002. The oncologist and my family had left the hospital. I wrote:

*"The Only Thing We Have to Fear is Fear Itself"*
*Franklin D. Roosevelt*

Monday, May 6, 2002

Day 4 in the hospital. I've had blood work daily, leg X-rays, lung X-rays, and I am to have a CAT scan, bone scan, and a bone biopsy. If anything, they should know what I DON'T have! I am pretty content today—knowing what I know. I feel better with more information that I found on the Net. I have a feeling this is going to be a hiccup in my life. But I do go in and out of fear/bravery. I fear a lot of things.

- I am afraid I won't get to see my grandchildren to the fullness of life.
- I am afraid Bill will have to grow old alone.
- I am afraid my family will have to suffer emotional distress.
- I am afraid that I won't make it five years.
- I am afraid of what I don't know.
- I m afraid I haven't done enough yet—and I won't get the chance.

Following the "I am afraid" entries were these four statements:

- I am not afraid to fight this.
- I am not afraid to die.
- I am not afraid of chemotherapy
- I am not afraid to let people care for me.

I proceeded to leave the hospital at the end of that week, and to prepare for a trip to my summer school experience. I had to put CML out of my mind and focus on the here and now in my life. I had a second summer session of schooling for my master in Pastoral Theology. So CML really went out of my mind.

I believe the depression did not hit until that August. It was after I had begun the miracle drug Gleevec and I experienced the side effects of the drug that I became angry. I had bone pain, face and body rash, the diarrhea, extreme and chronic fatigue. I had blistery rashes coming up on my leg, which was painful. I honestly believe that I was in denial until then. It was like I could put off dealing with the reality of cancer if I just went on with my life. The side effects make the cancer real. If you have none, you can ignore it; but if you *feel* the effects, it is like a nagging child constantly pulling on your skirt needing attention. The journal entry went like this:

Day Two of being pissed! Not my normal attitude, but here it is. And now what do I do with it? All the while, I have heard "Oh, you are such a woman of faith!" and "You are handling this diagnosis so well!" I don't feel so strong and I do not have much faith right now! I am pissed and that's that! This little pity party I am having has lots of questions like: Why me? Why now? What the hell did I do to deserve cancer? I started helping the church when Christina was five. I have been involved in building up the kingdom that long and this is what I get! If this is your new ministry you gave me God, give me a chance to say NO THANKS! I want to live to be 95. I want to grow old with Bill. I want to see my grandchildren have grandchildren like grandma did. I want, I need, I have to have a life!! Why Lord have you forsaken me? This whole thing stinks!

Fear can do incredible things to someone. I believe when I feel anger, it is a cover up for fear. It was several weeks before I wrote in the journal again. I just steeped in the fear and anger until I was tired of being there.

The other stages of grief were important to me as well. I think it pertinent to mention them here. I do believe I was in denial for two months, going on with life and ignoring the knocking spirit at the door. Somehow, I felt that maybe if I ignored him, he would go away, this dragon I affectionately called "Leukie." When it was obvious that he was here to stay, I decided to get angry. After the anger, came the bargaining: If God would take this cross from me, I would do his work for all of my life. Then the final stage: the complete acceptance of fate. Acceptance was the most difficult one. Upon acceptance came the relinquishing of control. Control had always been my MO. Funny thing,

*Your thoughts will become your destiny.*
*~Matthew Kelly*

the bargain that I made with God made sense to me after the acceptance. I think that there was probably a purpose to my having cancer. The next step of my faith journey would be to discover that purpose. What was it that Leukie and I were supposed to be about? What was our function in the world? I didn't know the answers to those questions, but I did know one thing: My suffering, fear and pain made no sense to me if it was not for a purpose to serve.

I heard a speaker at a conference that I attended a couple of years ago. His message was not a new one to me, but at the time that I heard it; I plucked it from his lips and buried it deep within the core of my heart and soul. Matthew Kelly's message is one that has resonated with me like no other. He said, "Your thoughts will become your character. Your character will become your destiny." I was not about to let cancer define me—but only in the way that I would determine. I would not give in to the anger, the blame, the resentment, and all those negative feelings that would eat up my time and energy. Rather, I must find a way to make it bring people to a level of faith or understanding their own purpose. My thoughts would be my own and not be fueled by the emotions that could destroy me, but be motivated by the sense of direction I was meant to go. Cancer would color every chapter of the life that remained. I could not control that. I might as well get my crayons out and decide what color those chapters would be.

# Chapter 6

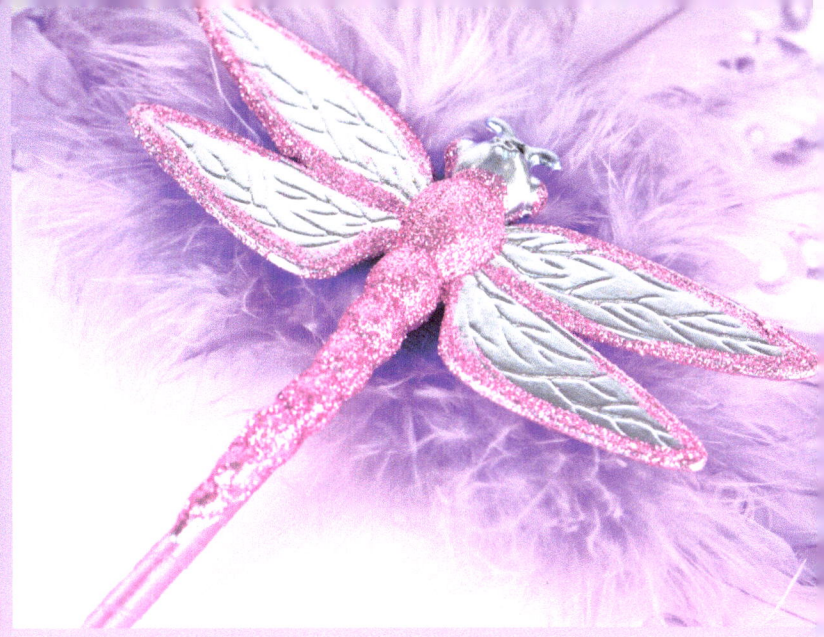

## KNOWLEDGE IS POWER

For me, knowledge was power. After the diagnosis, I began to read up on absolutely everything I could get my hands on. The bookcase was soon filled with books on leukemia, alternative healing, survivor stories, sad parables, and challenging tales. I began a diary of blood work numbers, prepared a binder with copies of all my tests, and recorded any and all pertinent information. I printed off all the information I could find on leukemia and shared all that information with anyone who might want it. I would compare each test to the other hoping to see some improvement in all of it. I learned more about leukemia than I ever in my life thought possible.

The City of Hope where I had consulted for possible transplant, invited us to their support group. I went for several weeks and discovered that these people were either pre- or post-bone-marrow-transplant patients. They invited me because I was investigating a transplant as an option. They met weekly and, as my knowledge grew about that option, I was relatively sure that I did not want to go that route if I didn't have to. Dr. Alvarnas had registered me for the National Bone Marrow Donor Program and they found two matches: eleven out of twelve antigens. They said I had "common linkages." My brother was tested and we found he was not a likely candidate to be my donor. Even Alvarnas said that we should give Gleevec a try before going into the transplant realm. I would have been a good candidate for him on which to try his new "mini-transplant" process. He was more interested in total care of me rather than his own interests. All of my doctors have been that way. I am so lucky.

Gleevec put me in remission at about nine months of drug therapy. I would begin to live this new chapter with one foot in the down side of side effects and the up side of PCRU—which means I was undetectable for the leukemia marker. Articles and books came out on the new miracle drug Gleevec. In reading about this new drug, I discovered that the Leukemia Lymphoma Society (LLS) had contributed financially to the research in the creation of this drug. I felt humbled. I also felt like I had to give back. There was no long-term data on Gleevec or projections of longevity. But for now, it had me in remission. I gathered up several folks that October and began what would be the first of many annual "Light the Night' walks. I raised about $2000 on my first walk. I was sent a banner named "Stanley Team," and folks carried it as we walked. Most of the walkers were support workers, caregivers, and people I call "do gooders" who carried the red balloon. Some of us carried the white "survivor" balloon. I remember the first walk. Several times during the walk, I looked up at the white balloons beside me and wanted to ask what disease they had—but I didn't. Several times, during the walk my eyes welled up and my throat was tight while I was filled with the emotions of gratefulness and hope. I was a survivor and not only could I survive because of these people, but I could help others survive. This would become one of the purposes of my having CML. Each year, I have been living with CML, I have participated in the LLS's Light the Night Walk. I now work each October with a group of students from our school in this endeavor. My husband has ever been at my side.

I began to attend a support group a few miles south of my house sponsored by LLS and held at a local hospital. It was meant for folks who had many different kinds of leukemia or lymphoma cancers. I was the only one with CML. I went for some time with my husband, but soon I decided that it was not the easiest thing to do. It seemed that, although we had similar cancers, I didn't feel like that was the place for me. I have never been able to put my finger on why. I felt almost guilty to be in remission while the rest of the group there struggled so hard to make it all come together for them. Another aspect was that it started at 6:30 in the evening. The rush to get home from school, eat, and fly to the meetings caused more stress in my life than was necessary. Others must have felt the same because they cancelled the group for a while because of low attendance.

The place I really found love and support, understanding, information was with Internet support groups. In this vastly developing technological world, the Internet was the best support I found. To this day, I actively engage in two on line groups, a chat group and several sites that give good and accurate information about blood cancers. I served in the capacity of a patient advisory board for a pharmaceutical company and most recently have the same position with the National CML Society. This position both keeps me informed and allows me to meet others who are on my journey. There is power in numbers and knowledge.

# Chapter 7

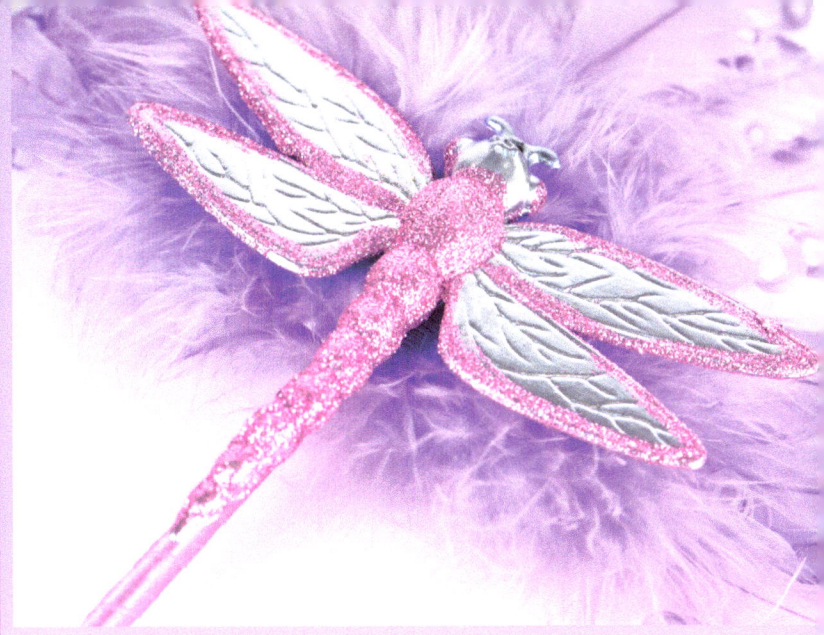

## THERE, BUT FOR THE GRACE OF GOD, GO I

There is an author that so eloquently put into words, the thoughts that became my daily mantra. Michael Learner said, "I would pay a great deal of attention to the inner healing process that I hope a cancer diagnosis would trigger in me. I would give careful thought to the meaning of my life, what I wanted to let go of and what I wanted to keep." This direction first popped into my head upon diagnosis. He goes on to say, "I would spend time with people I value and with books, writing music, and God. I would do everything I could do that I didn't want to leave undone."

The first thing that I want to share with you is how intentional life became. Now mind you, it wasn't over night, nor do I always live 100% in the way of which I am about to share. But it is my intention to move toward the way of life I describe, a small step at a time, for the rest of my life. I desire to do this because I believe it will bring me peace and healing.

*"It is never too late to become the person you were meant to be"*
*~ George Eliot*

My life should have intention. Two questions guided that intention:
1. What baggage do I carry around that keeps me from becoming the woman I am meant to be?
2. What can I find to do the rest of my life that will be congruent and harmonious with my inner self and my inner values?

I want to get up every morning with a purpose to what difference I might make that day. I believe I caused my own stress. I also believe that stress weakens our immune system and allows us to get sick. Am I saying that stress caused the cancer? I don't know. I have many theories about that. I am certain that stress causes high blood pressure and ill health. I do believe the way I lived my life added to the ability to get sick.

The old Barb would get up in the morning, pour coffee, look at the day timer, and see the many items that she must accomplish that day. She would eat on the run, run to work, run at work, run home, and run to another evening commitment only to fall in bed, pray for sleep, and rise the next day only to repeat the same pattern. I worked fifteen years in parish youth ministry. I worked all day from nine o'clock to five o'clock, preparing for family programs that would run from five o'clock to nine o'clock at night. I can't remember spending a Christmas Eve or an Easter with my family in fifteen years until I quit parish ministry. I moved down town to the Roman Catholic Diocese of Phoenix as an associate support staff in the Youth Ministry Office. My Day-Timer month-at-a-glance was filled with appointments, meetings, lunches, conferences, trips, consultations and in all, the more I had in the small daily squares, the more I felt important. Not only should they be daily accomplishments, but they should be done with perfection. There was no room for less. How sick is that?

I have lived in constant tension of balancing the home life with the work life. Talk to my two girls and I would guess they would tell you the home life got what was left over of me. That wasn't much. I know that our work in life should have meaning and mine did. But I do believe my work defined my life, my ego, and my self-identity—as professional. In past years, I am certain there was an addiction to work. The other identities of wife and mother, sister, daughter, aunt, and friend were at the bottom of that list. In these years, I also recognized the unhealthy way that I had manipulated my family. There, but for the grace of God went I! I hoped no one was watching!!

Then came cancer. It just reinforced at the time, that I was due for a change. I had been working on changing careers and was in the middle of the master degree. So at the time of diagnosis, I was in discernment with my spiritual director about which way I should look for a profession. I also was working in one of the unhealthiest environments I could imagine. I had recognized the feelings of it all, but cancer really helped me to define it. Looking back over my life, I can now see that each position or job I held taught me things about how to do the next one not only better, but with a little more intentional self care. If anything, I am grateful for CML as it is teaching me intentional self-care. I began to investigate a teaching position at a new school opening for the diocese. I got my substitute certificate, filled out the paper work, applied, and was accepted to the theology faculty at Notre Dame Preparatory High School in Scottsdale, Arizona. I am employed there today as theology department chair and I hope to retire from this institution. It really does provide an environment where I can live my values and fulfill my mission.

It was time to look at how I fed my own spirit. I instinctively knew that the things that would occupy my time should be things that feed me, my spirit, my emotions, and my wisdom. I had completed a two-year program that helped me to focus on youth at risk and their needs. The DeVoss Initiative helped me to assess my own life and goals. Out of that two-year process came my own mission statement that has guided my life ever since: "God has put me on this earth to create environments where people can be and become their very best." I began to see my role not as the "superwoman I-can-do-all-be-all-to-all," but more as a mentor and coach. I had learned those life lessons the hard way. Could I use them now to guide others? It gave my mistakes meaning and purpose. It gave me a sense of urgency to take really good care of myself for this second half of my life. Cancer only added fuel to that urgency.

Reflection was becoming an important part of my life. It was in the reflection that wisdom came fully. In that reflection, it became clear to me that I was out of control. Cancer would do what the cancer would do. I could take the medication and hope. But it would do what its own mind would tell it. Letting go has always been difficult. But in this letting go of the plans for my future, I could let go of the control I only thought I had over my life and look for the awareness of signposts along the way. That is not to say that I don't try to jump in behind the wheel of life and control it once again, but it has become less and less often. How freeing it is to let go! I began to focus more on what I could do while I was here on earth and not so much as what I could accomplish for myself. I began a deep desire to deepen my growth, physical, emotional, and spiritual. It would take time to create a practice in my life that would help me to do that.

God sent many people my way to help in my quest to be wise. Some were friends and some were family. Some were intentional and some not. But I am certain that the people who come into our lives come for a reason. Each person who enters my space is there to teach me something, to show me a mirrored refection to look at, to give me a comment, an idea, or a boost in the right direction. It became clear to me that this cancer diagnosis could help people become the best persons they could be if I used it correctly. This came to me early on in the cancer journey. As one entry in my journal says:

Lord, make me your instrument of grace. Take this affliction and make it a tool that glorifies your presence, and work in all the people I love. Help me to live by my mission, the mission I was given by you. Bring me an understanding of myself and the work you would have me do. Come Lord Jesus, come. Live in me and through me. But before you get started, would you take away my fear.

There are things much worse than a cancer diagnosis...

# Chapter 8

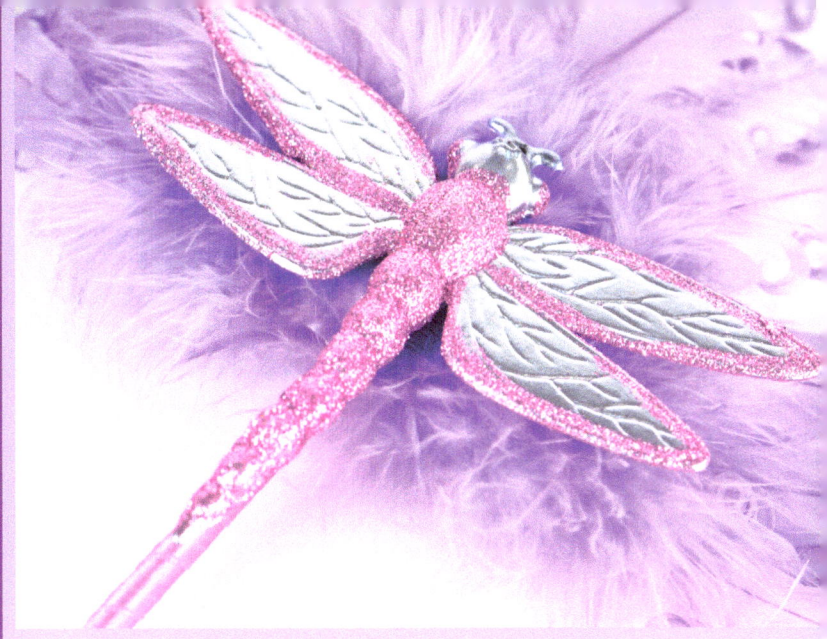

# THE ONGOING BUCKET LIST – SPIRIT FEEDING

At the onset of CML, I wrote down several goals that I had for sometime in the future. I remember breaking down in tears in a consultative office visit to the transplant doctor at City of Hope in Phoenix. He was giving me such hope at a time when I was so scared. I cried and told him, "I want to live!!" I think it was the only time that Bill ever saw me cry over the diagnosis. I am not sure whether that is a good thing or a bad thing. So what did I want to live for? I read a book called *If I Had My Life to Live Over* by Erma Bombeck. After much reflection, I wrote in my journal:

If I could live my life over again, these are the things I would want to do.
- I would have been more patient with my children when they were young.
- I would have spent more time with my grandmother.
- I would have gotten my degree sooner.
- I would have more patience with my husband.
- I would get up to see the sunrise once in a while.
- I would not take life so seriously, leave the house dirty once in a while and look the other way.
- I would spend much more time in solitude and with God.
- I would have more flowerbeds in my back yard.
- I would tell Bill and the children how proud of them I was and that I loved them *every day*.
- I would make sure I had fresh flowers every week.
- I would take more photos.
- I would learn how to play the piano.
- I would spend more time with my girlfriends.
- I would have challenged the things I disagreed with more.
- I would have walked in the woods more.

Reflection on this entry caused me to discover that there were only three top items I probably could not do at this time in my life. My grandma was gone, but she was with me in memory and spirit. My children were grown, but they were nearby. My degree could still be a reality. Outside of the first three regrets, every other item on my list was doable and RIGHT NOW!! It became clear to me that, if I put as much time and energy into living with no regrets, I could die a happy woman, no matter when that time came. If my mission and purpose for others was to create an environment where people could be and become their very best, why not do that for myself? Nothing beats a good role model.

The graduation from Saint Mary's University of Minnesota became my focus and reality. In May of 2004, I walked for the Master's hood. My family flew back to be with me at this joyous occasion. The degree became a reality.

Shortly after the diagnosis, a good friend came to me and asked me whether Bill and I would like to travel with them. I had met this woman in one of my parish positions. She was then and continues to be a woman who inspires me and a friend who makes me do things I wouldn't normally do. She broadens my world, my attitude, and my vision. She loves me for who I am and she makes me a better person for having her in my life. We traveled to Scotland for three weeks and visited Ireland with her and her husband. I am sad for the attitude I had to "rush to see all of it because I may not live long enough to come back." It put some stress on me being there; however, the trip is one memory that will forever be embedded in my heart.

More recently, I added to the bucket list a desire that people thought I was ridiculous. I fulfilled one item off the list when I rode in a NASCAR at 150 mph on the Phoenix racetrack. My daughter Christina went with me and together we made this memory. She had lit the fire of NASCAR racing several years ago. She is also a woman who makes me do fun things. She got me interested and almost fanatic about racing and now it is our shared addiction!

I added a return trip to Ireland. This trip is in the dreaming stages as I write. I am returning with a good friend of twenty years. She is someone who has once again, been by my side, believed in me, listened for hours on end when I needed to vent, asked me pertinent questions to cause self-reflection and, in all, experienced life almost in tandem with me. We were both from the Midwest, had husbands with similar interests, and we both entered ministry in the church in the diocese of Phoenix at the same time. She lost her mother first, and I followed her in losing mine. We shared the grief. We became grandparents three months apart and, in all, we really had tandem lives that spurred many a long discussion.

She and I and three other friends began to gather monthly for prayer, reflection, and fun. This group of five women soon became my "angel chick" group. They prayed over me, laid hands on me, lifted me in deep prayer, and I do believe began the healing process for me, both physically and spiritually. My angel prayer group feeds my spirit and my hope. I will continue to fulfill and add to my bucket list. Currently my bucket list includes ten items:

1.  Return to Ireland.
2.  Sky dive.
3.  Learn to drive a motorcycle.
4.  Travel to Jerusalem and Rome.
5.  Put in place a permanent schedule of intentional self-care every day.
6.  Take a trip with my two daughters to Europe.
7.  Write a book.
8.  Learn Yoga
9.  Build a garden in my back yard.
10. More to come!

# Chapter 9

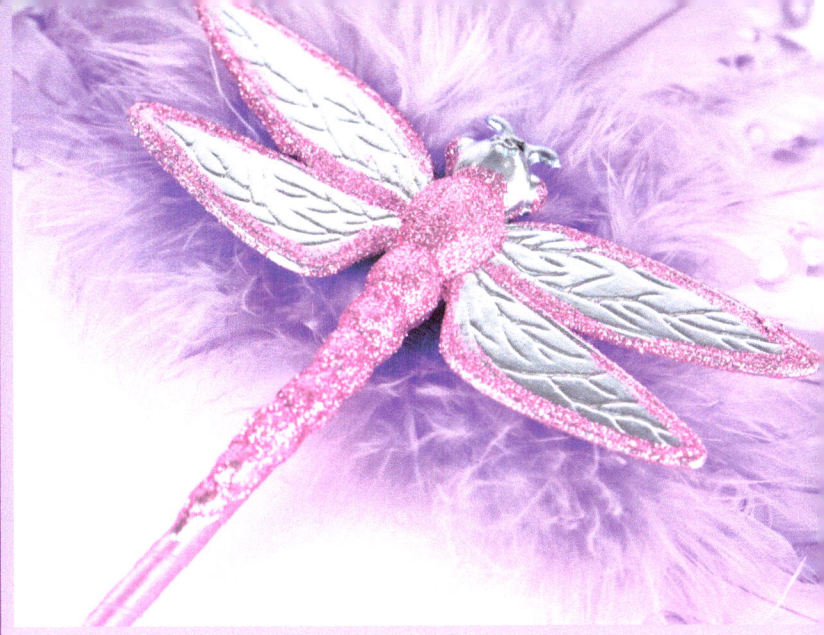

## RITUALS, SIGNS, AND SYMBOLS

## SIGN – Watch for the Signs...

In reflection on the past, there has been a lot of sign, symbol, and ritual of life for me. I connect the signs of our lives as synchronicity in our lives, karma, energies (if you will) that connect us to things, places, and people that were meant to be. You can explain them away as consequences of actions, but to me, they are signs, directives of how we are to follow—and they are only functional when we are aware of them. Otherwise, they pass us by, never to be connected as guides of the journey. Awareness is the key—and to cultivate awareness is my life's work.

In Red Oak, far ahead of my entrance to beauty school, a year before I went, a woman talked to me about a job if I needed one. I took this as a sign that I was supposed to go to beauty school. I can see now that, when the woman who owned the in-home beauty salon in Red Oak called me to see whether I wanted to buy her place, that was a sign for me to begin my own business. My husband losing his job in the middle of our discernment to move to Arizona was the sign that we were to go. My position being eliminated from the diocese was a sign that I should leave there and try another profession. The position being open at Notre Dame was another sign that I should apply. Leukemia, itself a sign, that I should prioritize my life—and do so with integrity. Many people find death in a moment's notice without time to do the important things that we need to do. An accident, a heart attack or a stroke seldom give people the time to say what they need to say, do what they need to do, or make their wrongs right before they leave the world. Cancer—CML—serves me as a sign at the end of a road that says "No Outlet"—in other words, there is no other path to take. This is a dead end. CML will always be with me. *But* I can turn around and find a different path for CML and me. I can take this lemon and make lemonade. I can make this affliction work in a positive way for me.

Signs are a grace to me, and if you define grace as God's loving presence, in fact, these signs become directional markers from God. I continue to be aware of the things in my life that provide direction for me. Sometimes I take the direction after the fact, but more often I take it during the event. But the key for me is being aware of the signs when they come, recognizing them for what they are, and in reflection, finding the meaning and the importance of them in my life. CML has given me *time* to reprioritize my life with integrity and with sacred intention.

## SYMBOL - Things Are Not Always What They Seem...

"Symbol," as defined by Wikipedia, is "something such as an object, picture, written word, sound, or particular mark that represents something else by association, resemblance, or convention." The Red Cross symbol is a universal sign of first aid or help. The stick figure of a man or woman communicates male and female bathrooms. The circular arrows indicate recycling. The stick figure in a half circle represents disabilities.

The cross I wear on my neck symbolizes and communicates to people I meet that I believe in Christianity. The wall of crosses I have collected on my dining room wall all communicate the same message. Other symbols in my life include the anniversary band my husband gave me for our thirtieth anniversary to mark our years together. Angels as a sign of spiritual guides for me have become very important in my life. I have angels on two walls in my home. I collect them. Most of my jewelry is gold. I have always resonated with it because of its resilience…"like gold tested in fire." It represents strength for me. I have a wall of family photos in my living room and they represent for me, stability. Below them, all is a wall appliqué that says, "Home is where our story begins." I have plants around my home that represent for me life.

CML is a symbol for me. It only takes the form of the Philadelphia chromosome in my blood, seen only under a microscope, but it is my symbol. It represents for me change and chance. It is a physical change from the ninth and twenty-second chromosome. It is a change in my health status. It is a change in the quality of my life when the side effects take the joy out of the day. Managing them is something that will be a daily task. It is a change in the medical routines that will require frequent blood testing, charts, and monitoring. It is also a chance: a chance of time. The original diagnosis could have been three to five years to live. Today, with modern medication, it is a chance to live my life different. That is the greatest gift of my cancer.

The most recent symbol to have meaning for me is the butterfly that I have tattooed on my left ankle. I did not do this as a youthful stunt in my teens. I did this for my forty-fifth birthday as a gift from my daughter who went with me. I had a purple and yellow butterfly tattooed because of its symbolism. My grandmother Catherine had always said that we were "becoming" all the time. She said that I was like a cocoon and butterfly. She told me that the first half of my life was the cocoon in which I worked hard to see what I would become. I was morphing into my future, busy as could be, and that work would produce who I would become. When the butterfly finally would emerge in the second half of my life, I could be beautiful as the butterfly. I could bring beauty to others as well. At forty-five years, it was time to look into the second half of my life and enjoy the work of the first half. To this day, butterflies and angels are my symbols at the front of my mind of each day.

## RITUAL – Actions Speak Louder Than Words…

We are all familiar with the rituals of life and easily recall the ones that have lined our histories. We blow out candles on birthday cakes. We open presents at Christmas time. We all have our personal morning rituals in the bathroom. Some folks have anxiety when their rituals are interrupted. People find comfort in consistency of ritual, its stability, and steadiness. That is why we all go to great measures to pack things for a trip that will keep order to our days.

In the case of having leukemia, the most important ritual for me was a Catholic sacrament of anointing of the sick. It used to be called the "Last Rites" and my understanding was that it was celebrated when people were close to death, a spiritual cleansing and healing to prepare them to meet God. Today, the church celebrates this sacrament as a healing sacrament, either physical or spiritual. While I was at the hospital on original diagnosis, the priest from our parish came to the hospital to anoint me—only to find out he could not. I had neutropenia; thus, people who entered my room needed masks and gloves to come in for fear I would pick up something my body couldn't fight. So he could not touch me. Instead, that sacrament was celebrated with my cohort at college in Winona, Minnesota, three weeks later. I can see now that was the place it was meant to be.

While at Saint Mary's University we had morning and evening prayer each day. It was held in a chapel that was located in our dorm. My neutropenia under control, I approached the Fr. Michael, one of our instructors, to ask whether I could be anointed at one of the evening prayer services. He spoke with the faculty and they all agreed that it would be fine. Two others wanted to receive the sacrament as well. Jack and John from the cohort both had health issues and asked to be included. That ceremony was, I believe, the turning point in my spiritual and physical healing. The ceremony included song, scripture, and ritual. The most powerful thing for me was the ritual. At a point in the anointing service, the priest came to lay hands on my head. Then he followed that with oil, anointing my forehead in the sign of the cross. As the oil ran down my face, he invited the community, one at a time, to come forward and lay hands on us also. If you believe in the adage that "there is power in numbers," I will tell you, "I am living proof." As each person came to lay his or her hands on my head and pray for my healing, a feeling of the presence of God absolutely overwhelmed me and moved me to uncontrollable sobbing. Those human hands laid on me individually and with prayer, reinforced for me, the message over and over, as if God were saying; "You will be healed. God's loving presence is with you. You will be healed." It remains for me, the most significant time that I have fully felt God's presence in my life.

Another significant ritual for me was one for which I had no plans. On Christmas Eve in December 2002, seven months after my diagnosis, I received a gift from my husband that, to this day, remains a daily reminder for me to "fight the good fight." Having been told on December 12 that I had reached molecular remission on this new drug, his gift to me was a license plate that reads: LEUKFRE. When I cried, my children said, "I guess she likes it, Dad." I did. The ritual of gift giving has taken on a whole new meaning for me. The sign of the license plate has people honking and waving at me on occasion, giving me the thumbs up through the windshield. What joy it gives me.

# Chapter 10

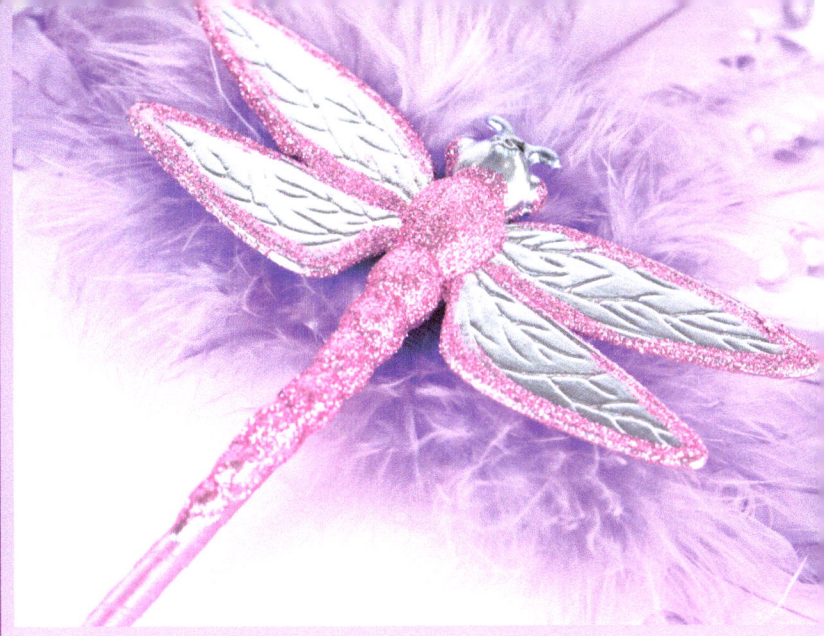

# WHEN THE STUDENT IS READY, THE TEACHER WILL COME

*L*ife gives us lessons to learn—if we recognize them as they appear. I am fairly sure that most of these lessons would have come to me at some time before I died. However, I am most grateful that I know them now. I think the grace of cancer has been that it moved the lessons up in my schedule of life. I believe that those lessons became more important when there became a risk of shortened life span. The awareness of brevity sparks a need to make sense of it all. What have I learned?

- I have thought often of the mistakes I made as a teenager, as a parent to my two beautiful girls, with my husband, in my work relationships, and friends. I could live each day in feeling regret, shame, self disappointment and depression, or I could reflect on those mistakes and identify what I could learn about myself, my choices and my life. I choose to do the latter. Whatever makes me a good person today is compiled from the experiences I have learned from in the past. I sincerely believe that mistakes are only opportunities to grow. Who I am today is a result of the choices I made. However, who I am becoming is a direct result of what I have done with them. It is no different with cancer. How I choose to react and respond to the illness, will make a difference in who I become with the time I have left.

- I have learned that I don't have to change friends or spouses, if I understand that friends and spouses change. I believe in the most intimate relationships that we have with our family and friends; we have to be patient with our growth patterns. I believe we all change, and if we can be accepting and supportive, then that change can and will enhance each person in the relationship.

- I am learning that it takes a long time to become the person whom I want to be. I am praying for a lot of patience from people who love me on this one. I might never get there!

- I have learned that I should always leave loved ones with loving words. It might be the last time I see them.

- I have learned that I can keep going long after I think I can't.

- I have learned that I must either control my attitude or it will control me. This is the hardest for me to work with because those old tapes that I keep in storage really don't understand the new gigabytes coming at them. It is difficult to change behavior patterns that have been long practiced.

- I have learned that I am responsible for my own happiness. No one in my life can make me happy. It is how I see the world, define my needs, and respond to them that makes my day or breaks it. I am in charge of that.

- I have learned that love is a choice: self-love and other love. The "in love" feeling goes away and it is work to get glimpses of that again.

- I have learned that my best friend and I can do anything or nothing, and have the best time.

- I have learned that I can have the right to be angry, but that doesn't give me the right to be cruel.

- I have learned that maturity has more to do with what I have done with the experiences I have had and less to do with how many years I have lived.
- I have learned that mistakes are opportunities to grow.
- I have learned that sometimes it isn't enough to be forgiven by others. Sometimes I have to learn to forgive myself.
- I have learned that my background and circumstances have influenced who I am, but that I am responsible for whom I become.
- I have learned that two people can look at the same thing and see it very different. That should be okay—all the time.  *CML was a good thing......*
- I have learned that, just because someone doesn't love me in the way I think they should, it doesn't mean they don't love me with all they have.
- I have learned that my life can be dramatically changed in a matter of hours by people who don't even know me.
- I have learned that reflection is an important part of our lives if life is to make sense.
- I have learned I am free when I let go and let God.

# Chapter 11

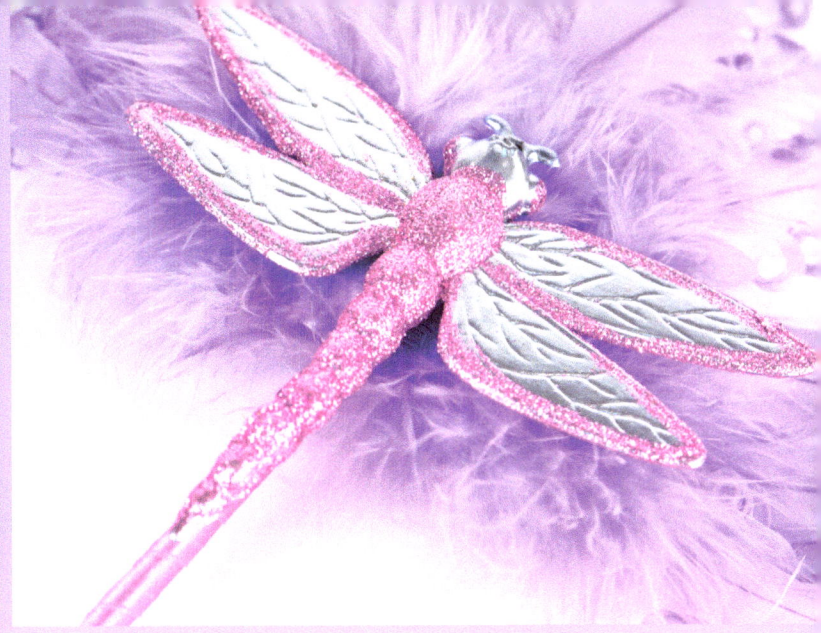

# THE WRITING IS ON THE WALL

In the closing chapter of this work, I would like to share with you what my diagnosis has done for me. I can't wish any cancer on anyone nor did I wish it on me. But the fact is that I have it. When I finally got to the stage where I could accept having this dreaded disease, I thought that I really needed to have this question answered for me: WHY me? In the depths of my grieving process over the loss of my good health, I cursed at God, asking this deity, "If this is the repayment for all the work I have done in *your* Name, it just doesn't make sense." I had worked for the church for fifteen years, helping teens and families to see the work of God in their lives. Was this what I should get in return?

This is where faith comes in. I have often said to people that I do not understand how people who have no faith deal with the loss of anything. If I could not believe that my loved ones were in a place where there was incredible peace and tranquility, their deaths would have no meaning to me. Also, if I could not believe that there is a purpose for my living with CML, it makes no sense for me to have it. If I truly believe my goal in life is to create a space where people can be and can become their very best, then CML has to fit in there somewhere. So how has having cancer improved my life and the life of others? That is what I want to share with you.

CML wasn't the best thing to have happened to me but it has proved to be a good thing. Maybe it is attitude and maybe it is simply hard work, but the truth is that it has improved the quality of my life. It has affected the way I think about the world. As my feet hit the floor each day, it has changed my motivation.

I have had the opportunity to help people believe in something greater than themselves, a higher power to order their lives. My strong testimony to the power of prayer is why my remission has been so strong. I often give credit to the remission to the people who pray for me and not necessarily the drugs. In reality, for me, I am sure that it is the combination of both; it is the prayer of the communion of saints, both living and dead, that have enabled me to continue my life with the quality I have. I can't explain why other people don't have the response to prayer that I have had, and I wish I could explain it, but for me, I am certain that it is a direct result of the power of prayer and faith. I tell the kids in my classroom that, if they have a hard time believing in miracles, I am living proof of them.

The cancer diagnosis has allowed me the opportunity of the time to reorder the important things in my life. My journey of life is a long one and it needs constant revising and editing to being me to the authenticity I want to live. Prior to the diagnosis, I think I tended to let my life run me instead of me running it. I think most of us do that. I also believe I might have gotten to this important lesson at some time in my life without cancer, but the diagnosis has moved it up on the lifelong "to do" list. It has given me the motivation to intentionally make choices that are good for my body, my mind, and my spirit. I live my life with more intention than I did before. I do self-care better than before, making sure that the choices I make are ones that will move me toward the person I want to become and as whom I want to be remembered. If it is true that we become our choices, I want my choices to be in sync with my inner self. If I could write on the wall of every bathroom in the hospital cancer wards, I would write the following message:

> Watch your thoughts; they become words. Watch your words; they become actions. Watch your actions; they become habits. Watch your habits; they become character. Watch your character; it becomes your destiny. (Anonymous)

This quote fits well into the morality class I teach, but it also fits into the lives of all of us and more so, for those of us with the possibility of a limited number of years. Cancer had given me the opportunity to look at and choose for myself, the way I take care of my body, what I put in it, how I treat it, exercise it and care for it. I have the opportunity to grow my mind with knowledge. I am an avid reader and gatherer of information on the Internet. I seldom go anywhere without my laptop. For me, knowledge is power. I have the opportunity to investigate and employ ways to feed my spirit that enhance my life and give me strength. Meditation has become an important part of my life, prayer groups, and prayer experiences and retreats all to enhance the spirit of life in me.

I have had the opportunity of the time to tell the people I love that I love them. I remember spending time with my mother three weeks before she passed away and, although our relationship in my younger years was tumulus, I was able to say to her the things to her I have always wanted to say. We seldom get the chance to say those things before we die. I felt like those three weeks were a gift, both for me and for her. So now, I try always to end the conversations with "I love you," so that, if these should be the last words they hear from me, they will know that I love them.

So in closing, the three purposes of my living with cancer, the things that I believe my cancer serves are (a) the ability to help others believe, (b) the ability to reorder my priorities and (c) the grace of time to tell people what they mean to me.

If I should be so bold as to offer advice to you, it would look like this:

- Learn as much as you can about your disease, cancer, or health situation. The more you know, the better equipped you are to make choices about your own health care and the direction you might go.
- Be involved in your health care. Don't leave it to the professionals (although they do a pretty good job). It has been proven that the more involved you are with your own health care, the better care you get.
- Take time to do an inventory and reflect on the important things in your life. Ask yourself what can you do that will make your world (that you are in charge of) a better place for you to live.
- Make a dream list or a "bucket list" to focus your energies on. The steps can be small steps, but at least you will be moving in a direction that will give you satisfaction.

- Learn about and implement good self-care. If this means setting boundaries for yourself, then so be it. You are the only one who can care for you.

In closing, I will finish the quote by Michael Lerner that I began earlier:

"I would give careful thought to choosing a mainstream oncologist. I wouldn't need someone with wonderful empathic skills because I have other people to provide that. But I would want a doctor who is basically kind, is on top of the medial literature regarding my disease, takes the time to answer my questions, understands that I want to be deeply involved in treatment decisions, supports my use of complimentary therapies and sticks with me medically and emotionally as if I were facing death. I would use conventional therapies that offered a real chance for recovery, but I would probably not use experimental therapies or therapies with low probability of success that were highly toxic or that would compromise my capacity to live and die as I might choose. I would use complimentary therapies, and I would look for a good support group and a psychotherapist experienced in working with people with cancer. I would look for ways to enhance my nutrition. I would meditate and practice yoga more often and spend more time in nature, walking in the woods, by the ocean and in the mountains. I would definitely try Chinese medicine, both herbs and acupuncture. I would strive for life and recovery with every possible tool and resource I could find. But I would also work to face death in a way that deepened my growth and led to some resolution. I would spend time with people I value and with books, writing, music, and God. I would so everything I could that I didn't want to leave undone. I would not waste time with old obligations although I would try to extricate myself from them decently. I would try to live my own life in my own way. I would try to accept the pain and the sorrow inherent in my situation, but I would look searchingly for the beauty, wisdom, and joy."

Also, a friend sent me this quote: "Please take this with the loving spirit in which it is sent and do with it what you will." I would concur with what she said.

I don't want to be remembered for how I died, but for how I lived.

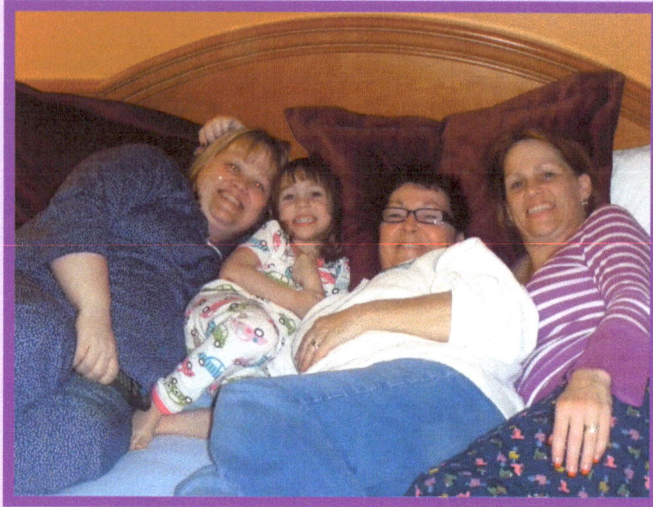

Grandma and her girls

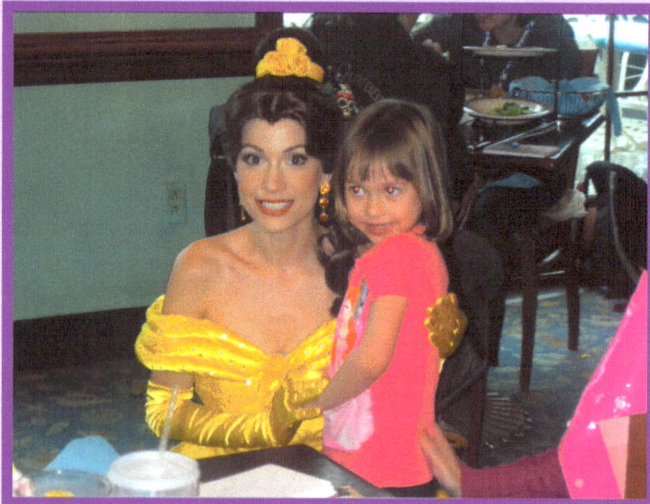

Mia and her favorite princess!

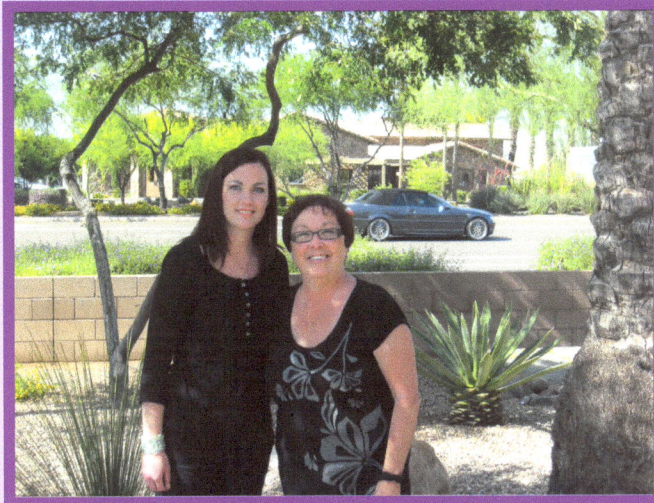

Gramma Barb and Dani

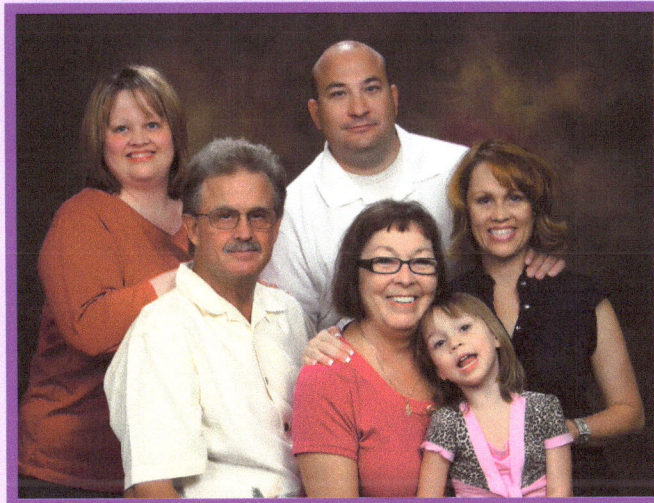

"The Family"

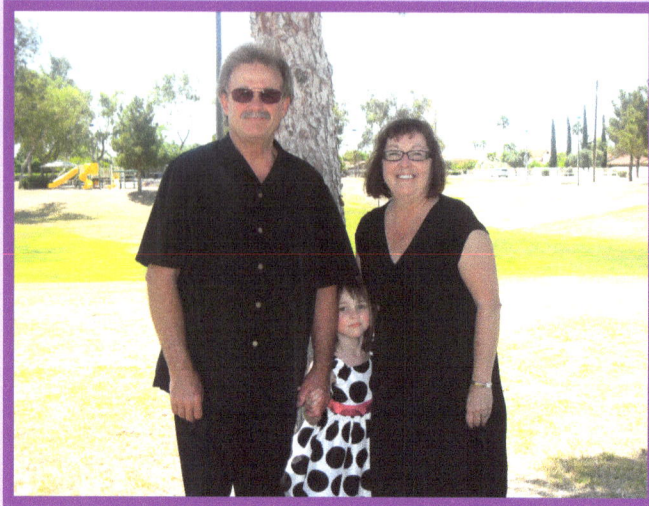

Grandma and Grandpa at Easter 2011

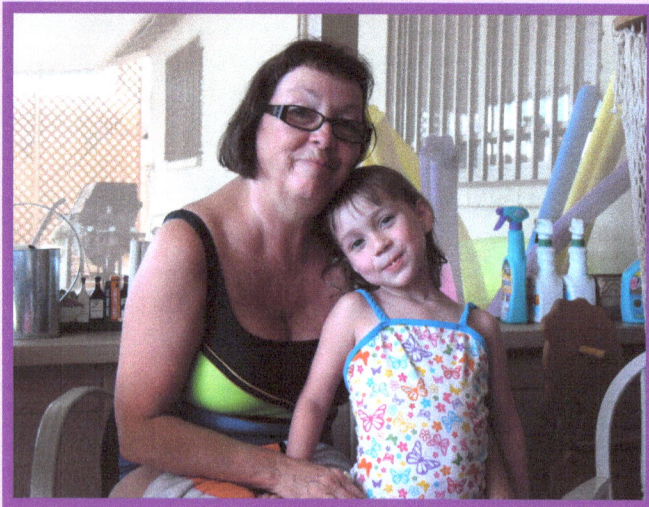

Happy Summer Days

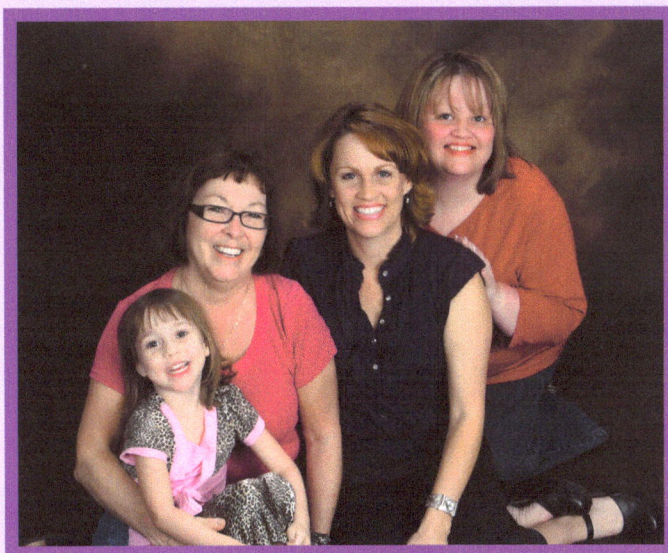

Angel Chicks

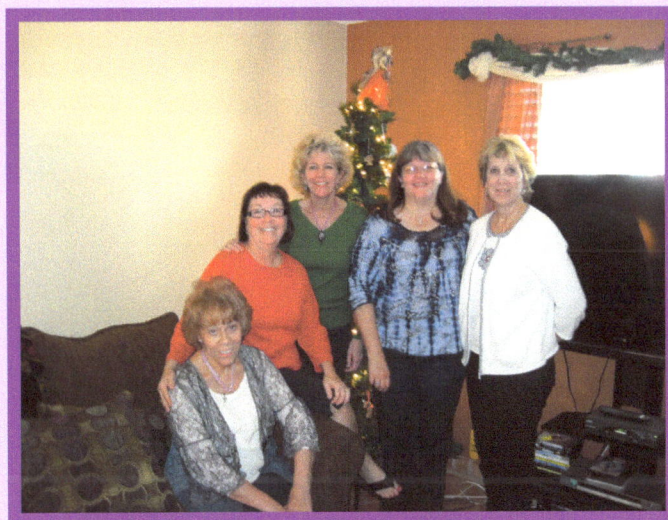

Holiday Angel Chicks

www.ingramcontent.com/pod-product-compliance
Lightning Source LLC
Chambersburg PA
CBHW060817270326

41930CB00002B/67